Hemodynamic Monitoring Study Guide

2nd Edition

D1368002

Dana Oakes

Scot Jones

DANA F. OAKES BA, RRT-NPS
Educational Consultant

Formerly:
Director of Clinical Education
Respiratory Care Program
Columbia Union College
Tacoma Park, Maryland

Educational Coordinator/Instructor
Respiratory Care Department
Children's Hospital Nat. Medical Center
Washington, D.C.

Director of Respiratory Care
VA Medical Center
Washington, D.C.

SCOT JONES BA, RRT-ACCS
Educational Consultant

Formerly:
Director of Clinical Education
Respiratory Care Program
Broward College
Coconut Creek, Florida

Respiratory Care Supervisor
Respiratory Care Department
Vidant Medical Center
Greenville, NC

ISBN 978-0-932887-04-7

2nd edition

RespiratoryBooks
A Division of Health Educator Publications, Inc.
476 Shotwell Road
Suite 102, PMB 161
Clayton, NC 27520

Important Disclaimer:

The Authors and Publisher has exerted every effort to ensure that the clinical principles, procedures, and practices described herein are based on current knowledge and state-of-the-art information available from acknowledged authorities, texts, and journals. Nevertheless, they cannot be considered absolute and universal recommendations. Each patient situation must be considered individually. The reader is urged to check the package inserts of drugs and disposable equipment and the manufacturer's manual of durable equipment for indications, contraindications, proper usage, warnings, and precautions before use. The Author and Publisher disclaim responsibility for any adverse effects resulting directly or indirectly from information presented in this book, undetected errors, or misunderstandings by the readers.

Table of Contents

Some Beginning Words

This study guide was designed to accompany the *Oakes' Hemodynamic Monitoring Pocket Guide*. It follows the pocket guide chapter-by-chapter with exercises that range from memorization (recall) to critical thinking.

For good reason we don't see the number of invasive lines in critical care units that we once saw. However, they still play a critical role in some patients. This actually makes this study guide that much more important as we need to make sure we are maintaining our knowledge levels.

This book has a couple different types of questions in it:

1. **Review Questions**
   Answers to these questions can be found in the back of the book
   There are a variety of types of questions meant to test your ability to recall and apply information. It is recommended that you work through these - look up any answers you don't know (using Oakes' Hemodynamic Monitoring Pocket Guide), as this will help you learn and retain information.
2. **Test Questions**
   Answers to these questions can be found in the back of the book
   It is recommended that you take these after working through the review questions. Do not use the book to look up these questions prior to taking it - treat it as a test. Once you correct it, you will know exactly what areas, if any, you need to work further on.
3. **Critical Thinking Questions**
   Answers to these questions must be requested - check respiratorybooks. com for details on how to get these (don't worry, they don't cost any money!). These questions help take you to that next level - applying the information in various ways, including scenarios. They are meant to be thought-provoking and guiding, where the process of answering the question is actually more important than the answer itself.

Why is it so important to master this stuff? If you work critical care in particular, there is little as important as understanding the hemodynamics of your patients, of how these are impacted by ventilation strategies, and how they are impacted by various diseases and illnesses.

Let's get started!

Match the following parameters with the appropriate definition.

	Parameter		Definition
_____	1.	Arterial oxygen tension	a. Difference between arterial and mixed venous oxygen tensions
_____	2.	Alveolar-arterial oxygen tension difference	b. Partial pressure of oxygen dissolved in the arterial blood
_____	3.	Arterial oxygen saturation	c. Partial pressure of carbon dioxide in mixed venous blood
_____	4.	Arterial oxygen content	d. Partial pressure of oxygen in alveoli
_____	5.	Fraction of inspired oxygen	e. Difference between arterial and mixed venous oxygen contents
_____	6.	Alveolar oxygen tension	f. Index of acidity or alkalinity of arterial blood
_____	7.	Arterial hydrogen ion concentration (pH)	g. Total amount of oxygen in arterial blood
_____	8.	Mixed venous carbon dioxide tension	h. Fraction of oxygen in inspired air
_____	9.	Aterio- (mixed) venous oxygen content difference	i. Percent of hemoglobin in arterial blood saturated with oxygen
_____	10.	Aterio- (mixed) venous oxygen tension difference	j. Partial pressure difference between oxygen in the alveoli and oxygen in arterial blood

Match the following parameters with the appropriate definition.

	Parameter		Definition
_____	11.	Aortic diastolic pressure	a. Mean blood pressure in left atrium
_____	12.	Systolic blood pressure	b. Mean blood pressure in the pulmonary capillaries
_____	13.	Central venous pressure	c. Blood pressure in right ventricle at end systole
_____	14.	Left atrial pressure	d. Diastolic blood pressure measured at base of the aorta
_____	15.	Left ventricular end-diastolic pressure	e. Mean pressure in right atrium
_____	16.	Mean pulmonary artery pressure	f. Pressure in left ventricle at end diastole
_____	17.	Pulmonary artery wedge pressure	g. Difference in arterial blood pressure between systolic and diastolic phases
_____	18.	Pulse pressure	h. Systemic arterial pressure during systole
_____	19.	Right ventricular end systolic pressure	i. Time-averaged pulmonary artery pressure
_____	20.	Right atrial pressure	j. Mean blood pressure in central veins and right atrium

Match the following parameters with the appropriate definition.

Parameter		Definition	
_____	21. Afterload	a.	Cardiac output expressed per body surface area
_____	22. Preload	b.	Work performed by left ventricle
_____	23. Contractility	c.	Total force opposing ventricular ejection
_____	24. Stroke volume	d.	Measure of ventircular performance
_____	25. Cardiac output	e.	Percentage of ventricular chamber emptying
_____	26. Cardiac index	f.	Amount of blood ejected by either venticle per contraction
_____	27. Stroke work	g.	Myocardial fiber length at end diastole
_____	28. Ejection fraction	h.	Amount of blood pumped by the heart per minute
_____	29. Left ventricular stroke work	i.	Work performed by right ventricle per body surface area
_____	30. Right ventricular stroke work index	j.	Force of ventricle contraction independent of preload or after-load

Match the following parameters with the appropriate definition.

	Parameter		Definition
_____	31. Coronary perfusion pressure	a.	Quantity of oxygen pumped by the heart to body tissue per unit time
_____	32. Myocardial oxygen consumption (demand)	b.	Amount of oxygen delivered to the heart by coronary vessels
_____	33. Myocardial oxygen delivery (supply)	c.	Driving pressure of coronary blood flow
_____	34. Oxygen consumption index	d.	Venous oxygen supply
_____	35. Oxygen delivery	e.	Oxygen consumption per body size
_____	36. Oxygen extraction ratio	f.	Resistance to right ventircular ejection of blood into the pulmonary vasculature
_____	37. Oxygen reserve	g.	Plot reflecting cardiac output to left ventricular preload
_____	38. Pulmonary vascular resistance	h.	Amount of oxygen extracted and consumed by the body tissues relative to the amount of oxygen delivered
_____	39. Physiologic shunt	i.	Amount of oxygen consumed by the heart per minute
_____	40. Left ventricular function curve	j.	Percent of cardiac output which passes from the right atrium to the left atrium without being oxygenated

Match the following parameters with the appropriate definition.

Parameter		Definition	
_____	41. A-a DO$_2$	a.	Arterial oxygen saturation
_____	42. PAO$_2$	b.	Alveolar oxygen tension
_____	43. S$\bar{V}$O$_2$	c.	Arterio-(mixed) venous oxygen content difference
_____	44. CaO$_2$	d.	Mixed venous oxygen content
_____	45. Ca-$\bar{V}$ O$_2$	e.	Fraction of inspired oxygen
_____	46. a-$\bar{V}$ DO$_2$	f.	Alveolar-Arterial oxygen tension difference
_____	47. C$\bar{V}$O$_2$	g.	Arterio-(mixed) venous oxygen tension difference
_____	48. SaO$_2$	h.	Mixed venous oxygen saturation
_____	49 F$_1$O$_2$	i.	Arterial oxygen tension
_____	50. PaO$_2$	j.	Arterial oxygen content

Match the following parameters with the appropriate definition.

	Parameter		Definition
_____	51. $\dot{D}O_2$	a.	Oxygen extraction ratio
_____	52. $\dot{V}O_2$	b.	Oxygen consumption (demand)
_____	53. O_2ER	c.	Oxygen delivery index
_____	54. $M\dot{D}O_2$	d.	Oxygen delivery (supply or transport)
_____	55. $M\dot{V}O_2$	e.	Myocardial oxygen consumption (demand)
_____	56. $\dot{D}O_2I$	f.	Myocardial oxygen delivery (supply)
_____	57. $\dot{V}O_2I$	g.	Oxygen consumption index

Match the following parameters with the appropriate definition.

	Parameter		Definition
_____	58. BPsys	a.	Mean arterial pressure
_____	59. LVEDP	b.	Pulmonary artery pressure
_____	60. CVP	c.	Left atrial pressure
_____	61. MAP	d.	Pulmonary artery mean pressure
_____	62. PAMP	e.	Left ventricular end-diastolic pressure
_____	63. LAP	f.	Right ventricular end-diastolic pressure
_____	64. PAEDP	g.	Left ventricular end systolic volume
_____	65. PAP	h.	Systolic blood pressure
_____	66. LVESV	i.	Central venous pressure
_____	67. RVEDP	j.	Pulmonary artery end-diastolic pressure

Match the following parameters with the appropriate definition.

	Parameter		Definition
_____	68. AoD	a.	Pulmonary vascular resistance index
_____	69. CI	b.	Heart rate
_____	70. EF	c.	Aortic diastolic pressure
_____	71. BSA	d.	Stroke volume
_____	72. HR	e.	Cardiac index
_____	73. LVSW	f.	Cardiac output
_____	74. PVRI	g.	Pulse pressure
_____	75. CO	h.	Body surface area
_____	76. PP	i.	Left ventricular stroke work
_____	77. SV	j.	Ejection fraction

Put the letter of the normal value next to the numbered parameter.

	Parameter		Definition
_____	78. PAO_2	a.	15-24 mL/dL
_____	79. $P\bar{v}O_2$	b.	60 mm Hg
_____	80. CaO_2	c.	35-42 mm Hg
_____	81. SaO_2	d.	100 mm Hg
_____	82. $a\text{-}\bar{v}DO_2$	e.	95-100%
_____	83. P_{50}	f.	12-15 mL/dL
_____	84. $Ca\text{-}\bar{v}O_2$	g.	4.2-5.0 mL/dL
_____	85. $C\bar{v}O_2$	h.	27 mm Hg
_____	86. PaO_2	i.	75%
_____	87. $S\bar{v}O_2$	j.	80-100 mm Hg

Put the letter of the normal value next to the numbered parameter.

	Parameter		Definition
_____	88. $PaCO_2$	a.	46 mm Hg
_____	89. $P\overline{v}CO_2$	b.	750 - 1000 mL/min
_____	90. $PvCO_2$	c.	25%
_____	91. pHa	d.	35-45 mm Hg
_____	92. pHv	e.	0.21-100
_____	93. $\dot{D}O_2$	f.	200-250 mL/min
_____	94. $\dot{V}O_2$	g.	< 5%
_____	95. O_2ER	h.	7.40
_____	96. FIO_2	i.	7.36
_____	97. $\dot{Q}s/\dot{Q}t$	j.	Variable

Put the letter of the normal value next to the numbered parameter.

	Parameter		Definition
_____	98. BPsys	a.	0-6 mm Hg
_____	99. BPdia	b.	4-12 mm Hg
_____	100. MAP	c.	8-15 mm Hg
_____	101. PP	d.	10-15 mm Hg
_____	102. CVP	e.	15-25 mm Hg
_____	103. PASP	f.	40 (20-80) mm Hg
_____	104. PADP	g.	60-80 mm Hg
_____	105. PAMP	h.	70-105 mm Hg
_____	106. PAWP	i.	100-140 mm Hg

Put the letter of the normal value next to the numbered parameter.

	Parameter		Definition
_____	107. CO	a.	0-6 mm Hg
_____	108. CI	b.	4-12 mm Hg
_____	109. HR	c.	15-25 mm Hg
_____	110. SV	d.	100-140 mm Hg
_____	111. RAP	e.	4-8 L/min
_____	112. RVESP	f.	2.5-4.4 L/min/m²
_____	113. LAP (LVEDP)	g.	60-120 mL/beat
_____	114. LVESP	h.	60-100 beats/min
_____	115. PVR	i.	20-200 dynes•sec•cm^{-5}
_____	116. SVR	j.	800-1600 dynes•sec•cm^{-5}

Put the letter of the equation next to the numbered parameter.

	Parameter		Definition
_____	117. PaO_2	a.	$PaO_2 - P\bar{v}O_2$
_____	118. $A\text{-}aDO_2$	b.	$CaO_2 - C\bar{v}O_2$
_____	119. $a\text{-}\bar{v}DO_2$	c.	$PAO_2 - PaO_2$
_____	120. CaO_2	d.	$CO \times CaO_2 \times 10$
_____	121. $C\bar{v}O_2$	e.	$CO \times Ca - \bar{v}O_2 \times 10$
_____	122. $Ca\text{-}\bar{v}O_2$	f.	$SaO_2 - VO_2 / \dot{D}O_2$
_____	123. $S\bar{v}O_2$	g.	$\dot{V}O_2 / \dot{D}O_2 \times 100$
_____	124. $\dot{V}O_2$	h.	$[(Pb - PH_2O) FIO_2] - PaCO_2 \times 1.25$
_____	125. $\dot{D}O_2$	i.	$(SaO_2 \times Hgb \times 1.36)\ (PaO_2 \times 0.0031)$
_____	126. O_2ER	j.	$(S\bar{v}O_2 \times Hgb \times 1.36) + (P\bar{v}O_2 \times 0.0031)$

Put the letter of the equation next to the numbered parameter.

Parameter		Definition
_____ 127.	MAP (BP)	a. $CO \times CaO_2 \times 10$
_____ 128.	PP	b. $CO \times Ca - \bar{v}O_2 \times 10$
_____ 129.	CO	c. $BP_{sys} - BP_{dia}$
_____ 130.	CI	d. $(BP_{sys} + 2BP_{dia}) / 3$
_____ 131.	RVSW	e. $SV \times (PAMP - CVP) \times 0.0136$
_____ 132.	LVSW	f. $SV \times (\overline{BP} - PAWP) \times 0.0136$
_____ 133.	$\dot{V}O_2$	g. $HR \times SV$
_____ 134.	$\dot{D}O_2$	h. $[(\overline{BP} - CVP) \times 80] / CO$
_____ 135.	SVR	i. $[(PAMP - PAWP) \times 80] / CO$
_____ 136.	PVR	j. CO / BSA

Select the appropriate parameter for the following definitions

1. The partial pressure of oxygen dissolved in the arterial blood:
   a. Arterial oxygen content
   b. Arterial oxygen saturation
   c. Arterial oxygen tension
   d. Arterial oxygen tension difference

2. The mean blood pressure in the pulmonary capillaries:
   a. Pulmonary artery pressure
   b. Pulmonary artery wedge pressure
   c. Pulmonary capillary pressure
   d. Pulmonary capillary wedge pressure

3. The work performed by the left ventricle:
   a. Stroke work
   b. Cardiac Output
   c. Left ventricular stroke work
   d. Left ventricular cardiac output

4. The myocardial fiber length at end diastole:
   a. Preload
   b. Afterload
   c. Contractility
   d. Stroke work index

5. The percent of cardiac output which passes from the right atrium to the left atrium without being oxygenated:
   a. Cardiac Index
   b. Oxygen reserve
   c. Oxygen extraction ratio
   d. Physiologic shunt

6. Alveolar-arterial oxygen tension difference:
   a. a-$(\overline{v})DO_2$
   b. $Ca-\overline{v}O_2$
   c. $A-aDO_2$
   d. $Ca-AO_2$

7. Oxygen consumption:
   a. $\dot{D}O_2$
   b. $\dot{V}O_2$
   c. CO_2
   d. O_2ER

8. Oxygen demand:
   a. $\dot{D}O_2$
   b. $\dot{V}O_2$
   c. CO_2
   d. O_2ER

9. Oxygen delivery index:
   a. $\dot{D}O_2I$
   b. $\dot{V}O_2I$
   c. O_2ER
   d. O_2DI

	Parameter		Definition
_____	10. $A-aDO_2$	a.	arterial oxygen content
_____	11. PaO_2	b.	cardiac index
_____	12. $\dot{V}O_2I$	c.	oxygen delivery
_____	13. $a-\overline{v}DO_2$	d.	arterial oxygen tension
_____	14. CI	e.	alveolar-arterial oxygen tension difference
_____	15. FIO_2	f.	arterio-mixed venous oxygen tension difference
_____	16. CaO_2	g.	mixed venous carbon dioxide tension
_____	17. $P\overline{v}CO_2$	h.	oxygen consumption index
_____	18. MvO_2	i.	fraction of inspired oxygen
_____	19. $\dot{D}O_2$	j.	myocardial oxygen consumption

Select the normal value for the following parameters (#20-29)

20. Alveolar oxygen tension:
    a. 75 mm Hg
    b. 80-100 mm Hg
    c. 100 mm Hg
    d. 210 mm Hg

21. Arterial oxygen content:
    a. 4.2 – 5.0 mL/dL
    b. 12 – 15 mL/dL
    c. 15 – 24 mL/dL
    d. 80 -100 mL/dL

22. Arterio-(mixed) venous oxygen tension differences:
    a. 60 mm Hg
    b. 75 mm Hg
    c. 80 mm Hg
    d. 100 mmHg

23. Mixed venous carbon dioxide tension:
    a. 27 mm Hg
    b. 35 – 45 mm Hg
    c. 46 mm Hg
    d. variable

24. Oxygen delivery:
    a. 200-250 mL/min
    b. 750 -1000 mL/min
    c. 12 – 15 mL/min
    d. 15 – 24 mL/min

25. Pulmonary artery systolic pressure:
    a. 4 – 12 mm Hg
    b. 8 – 15 mm Hg
    c. 15 – 25 mm Hg
    d. 60 – 80 mm Hg

26. Mean arterial pressure:
    a. 40 mm Hg
    b. 60 – 80 mm Hg
    c. 70 – 105 mm Hg
    d. 100 – 140 mm Hg

27. Stroke volume:
    a. 60 – 100 mL/beat
    b. 60 – 120 mL/beat
    c. 2.5 – 4.4 L/min
    d. 8 – 12 L/min

28. Pulmonary vascular resistance:
    a. 20 – 200 dynes•sec•cm^{-5}
    b. 60 – 100 dynes•sec•cm^{-5}
    c. 100 – 140 dynes•sec•cm^{-5}
    d. 1200 – 1600 dynes•sec•cm^{-5}

29. Cardiac index:
    a. 15 – 25 L/min/m^2
    b. 4 – 8 L/min/m^2
    c. 4.2 – 5.0 L/min/m^2
    d. 2.5 – 4.4 L/min/m^2

Select the appropriate equation for the following parameters
30. Alveolar oxygen tension:
    a. $PAO_2 - PaO_2$
    b. $CO \times CaO_2 \times 10$
    c. $(SaO_2 \times Hgb \times 1.36) + (PaO_2 \times 0.0031)$
    d. $[(P_B - PH_2O) FIO_2] - PaCO_2 \times 1.25$

31. Arterial oxygen content:
    a. $CAO_2 - C\overline{V}O_2$
    b. $CO \times CaO_2 \times 10$
    c. $[(P_B - PH_2O)FIO_2] + PaO_2 \times 1.25$
    d. $(SaO_2 \times Hgb \times 1.36) + (PaO_2 \times 0.0031)$

32. Oxygen delivery:
    a. $CAO_2 - C\overline{V}O_2$
    b. $CO \times CaO_2 \times 10$
    c. $CO \times Ca - \overline{V}O_2 \times 10$
    d. $VO_2 / DO_2 \times 100$

33. Systemic vascular resistance:
    a. $CO \times BSA$
    b. $\overline{[(BP - CVP) \times 80]} / CO$
    c. $(BPsys - 2\ BPdia) / 3$
    d. $SV \overline{\times (BP} - PAWP) \times 0.0136$

34. Pulse pressure:
    a. BPsys - BPdia
    b. (BPsys + 2 BPdia) / 3
    c. SV x ($\overline{BP}$ - PAWP) x 0.0136
    d. HR x SV

	Parameter	Definition
_____	35. PaO_2 - $P\overline{v}O_2$	a. 25%
_____	36. CO x Ca - $\overline{v}O_2$ x 10	b. Variable
_____	37. SV x ($\overline{BP}$ - PAWP) x 0.0136	c. 20-200 dynes-sec-cm-5
_____	38. HR x SV	d. 60 mm Hg
_____	39. $\dot{V}O_2$ / $\dot{D}O_2$ x 100	e. 4.2 - 5.0 mL/dL
_____	40. [(PAMP - PAWP) x 80] / CO	f. 200 - 250 mL/min
_____	41. PAO_2 - PaO_2	g. 60-80 gm/m/beat
_____	42. BPsys - BPdia	h. 10 - 25 mm Hg
_____	43. SaO_2 - $\dot{V}O_2$ / $\dot{D}O_2$	i. 4 - 8 L/min
_____	44. CaO_2 - $C\overline{v}O_2$	j. 15 - 24 mL/dL
_____	45. (SaO_2 x Hgb x 1.36) + (PaO_2 x 0.0031)	k. 40 mm Hg

True or False:

_____ 46. Aortic diastolic pressure equals the mean BP at the root of the aorta

_____ 47. The normal value of central venous pressure is 0-8 cm H_2O

_____ 48. The normal ejection fraction is 65%

_____ 49. Normal LVEDP is 4-12 mm Hg

_____ 50. A left ventricular function curve is a plot reflecting CO-to-LV preload

1. There are often both noninvasive and invasive options for obtaining hemo-dynamic information on a patient. Explain the benefits and concerns of using noninvasive versus invasive options?

2. A 31-year-old woman is admitted to the ICU with suspected septic shock, and is requiring mechanical ventilation with frequent ABGs ordered. BP is currently 74/46.
    a. Which invasive lines are indicated?

    b. What is her mean blood pressure? How should this blood pressure be classified?

    c. Explain the physiologic meaning of the blood pressure in b (what spe-cifically is happening with body functions at this pressure?).

3. Complete the following. This will be a good tool for you later on, so it is recommended that you use different colors for anatomy versus parameters.

   a. Draw and label a diagram of the heart (it does not have to be anatomically correct, but it should be representative of the key anatomy).

Left Atrium	Aortic Valve	Aorta
Left Ventricle	Mitral Valve	Inferior Vena Cava
Right Atrium	Pulmonary Valve	Pulmonary Artery
Right Ventricle	Tricuspid Valve	Superior Vena Cava

   b. Now, using the diagram you drew, place each of the below listed parameters in the portion(s) of the heart being measured (what is directly measured or what is indirectly being reflected in the measurement):

CVP	LVEDV	RAP
EF	PAP	RVEDP
LAP	PAWP	RVEDV
LVEDP	PVR	SVR

1. The cardiopulmonary system's primary purpose is the delivery of (a)
   _____ and (b) _____at a rate

   (c)_____. The ultimate goal is

   (d) _____.

For the following, indicate whether the parameter is most likely to INCREASE or DECREASE during decreased (inadequate) tissue perfusion:

2. _____ Heart rate

3. _____ Arterial pulse

4. _____ Pulse pressure

5. _____ Respiratory rate

6. _____ Urinary output

7. _____ Level of Consciousness

8. _____ Skin temperature

9. _____ Capillary refill (time)

10. The quantity of O_2 pumped by the heart to the body tissues per unit time is:
    a. O_2 supply
    b. O_2 demand
    c. O_2 reserve
    d. O_2 consumption

11. The quantity of O_2 utilized by the body tissues per unit time is:
    a. O_2 supply
    b. O_2 demand
    c. O_2 reserve
    d. O_2 delivery

12. O_2 reserve equals:
    a. Arterial O_2 supply
    b. Venous O_2 supply
    c. Tissue O_2 supply
    d. Capillary O_2 supply

13. Which of the following is true?
    a. O_2 Reserve = O_2 Supply + O_2 Demand
    b. O_2 Reserve = O_2 Supply - O_2 Demand
    c. O_2 Reserve = O_2 Consumption + O_2 Delivery
    d. O_2 Reserve = O_2 Consumption - O_2 Delivery

14. Normal O_2 supply is:
    a. 250 mL/min
    b. 750 mL/min
    c. 1000 mL/min
    d. 1250 mL/min

15. Normal O_2 reserve is:
    a. 250 mL/min
    b. 750 mL/min
    c. 1000 mL/min
    d. 1250 mL/min

16. Normal O_2 demand is:
    a. 250 mL/min
    b. 750 mL/min
    c. 1000 mL/min
    d. 1250 mL/min

17. The body's first response to an increase in tissue O_2 demand is:
    a. An increase in anaerobic metabolism
    b. A decrease in O_2 reserve
    c. An increase in O_2 reserve
    d. An increase in O_2 supply

Match the following heart and pulmonary pressure waveforms:

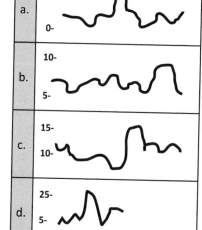

18. _____ Right atrium

19. _____ Right ventricle

20. _____ Left ventricle

21. _____ Pulmonary artery

22. _____ Pulmonary wedge

23. _____ Aorta

24. The a wave in a heart pressure waveform represents:
    a. A fall in pressure during atrial emptying
    b. A rise in pressure during atrial filling
    c. A fall in pressure during ventricular emptying
    d. A rise in pressure during ventircular filling

Place the following phases of the cardiac cycle in sequence.

Ventricular Systole

25. _____

26. _____

27. _____

Ventricular diastole

28. _____

29. _____

30. _____

a.   Passive filling

b.   Reduced ejection

c.   Isovolumetric relaxation

d.   Isovolumetric contraction

e.   Atrial systole

f.   Rapid ejection

Indicate whether the following factors affect myocardial oxygen supply ($M\dot{D}O_2$) or myocardial oxygen demand (MvO_2):

31. _____ Wall tension

32. _____ CaO_2

33. _____ Contractility

34. _____ Heart rate

35. _____ Coronary blood flow

Answer the following questions about CPP as True or False

36. _____ CPP stands for *Coronary Perfusion Pressure*

37. _____ CPP = AoD - Coronary Venous Pressure

38. _____ CPP = BPdia - LVESP

39. _____ CPP can be estimated: BPdia - PAWP

40. _____ The normal range of CPP is 60-80 mm Hg

Indicate whether the following are most representative of Cardiac Output (CO) and Cardiac Index (CI)

41. _____ BP = SVR x _____

42. _____ HR x SV = _____

43. _____ 2.5 - 4.2 L/min/m² = _____

44. _____ 4 - 8 L/min = _____

45. _____ The better indicator of circulatory status = _____

Answer the following as either True (T) or False (F)

_____ 46. The upstroke on an arterial blood pressure waveform is called the *dicrotic limb*

_____ 47. The most rapid and effective way to increase cardiac output is to increase heart rate

_____ 48. Stroke Volume = ESV - EDV

_____ 49. Preload is the end-diastolic muscle fiber length

_____ 50. Starling's Law states that the more the heart is filled (preload), the greater the contractile force (SV), within limits

_____ 51. A ventricular function curve represents the relationship between preload and heart rate

_____ 52. Ventricular function curves are used to determine optimal ventricular function and optimal PAWP

_____ 53. Afterload is the total force of ventricular ejection

_____ 54. The primary determinant of afterload resistance is arteriole wall tension

_____ 55. A clinical measure of LV afterload is BPdia + SVR

_____ 56. Afterload is directly proportional to stroke volume

_____ 57. Afterload is directly proportional to MvO_2

_____ 58. Afterload is the most important determinant of MvO_2

_____ 59. Contractility is the inotropic state of the pericardium

_____ 60. Contractility is inversely proportional to ventricular work

_____ 61. Changes in contractility are usually initiated by intrinsic factors

_____ 62. Systemic vascular resistance is the force the RV must overcome to maintain systemic blood flow

_____ 63. SVR = [(BP - CVP) / CO] x 80

_____ 64. Normal SVR = 800-1600 mm Hg/L/min

_____ 65. The primary determinant of SVR is arteriole diameter

_____ 66. The four main factors which regulate SVR are blood vessel diameter, blood volume, blood viscosity, and the kidneys

_____ 67. LV afterload is directly proportional to SVR

_____ 68. PVR is the force the RV must overcome to maintain pulmonary blood flow

_____ 69. PVR = $\dfrac{PAP - PAWP}{CO}$ x 80

_____ 70. Normal PVR = 20-200 dynes•sec•cm^{-5}

_____ 71. Oxygen is a potent vasoconstrictor of the pulmonary vessels

_____ 72. Pulmonary vasodilators act to increase pulmonary vascular resistance

_____ 73. RV afterload is directly proportional to PVR

1. The quantity of Oxygen pumped by the heart to the body tissues per unit time is:
    a. O_2 supply
    b. O_2 delivery
    c. O_2 transport
    d. All of the above

2. O_2 supply is a function of:
    a. Arterial O_2 tension - $P\overline{V}O_2$
    b. Arterial O_2 content - $C\overline{V}O_2$
    c. Arterial O_2 content x CO
    d. Arterial O_2 content / CO

3. O_2 reserve equals:
    a. O_2 supply + O_2 demand
    b. O_2 supply - O_2 demand
    c. O_2 supply / O_2 demand
    d. O_2 supply x O_2 demand

4. The Body's first response to an increase in tissue O_2 demand is:
    a. Decreased O_2 reserve
    b. Ventilatory failure
    c. Anaerobic metabolism
    d. Increased O_2 supply

5. The Body's second response to an increase in tissue O_2 demand is:
    a. Decreased O_2 reserve
    b. Ventilatory failure
    c. Anaerobic metabolism
    d. Increased O_2 supply

6. The Body's third response to an increase in tissue O_2 demand is:
    a. Decreased O_2 reserve
    b. Ventilatory failure
    c. Anaerobic metabolism
    d. Increased O_2 supply

Match the following

		Parameter		Definition
_____	7.	O₂ consumption	a.	25%
_____	8.	O₂ reserve	b.	250 mL/min
_____	9.	O₂ extraction ratio	c.	750 mL/min
_____	10.	O₂ supply	d.	1000 mL/min

Match the following parameters to their normal value range. Note that some ranges will be used more than once

		Parameter		Normal Range
_____	11.	$\overline{RAP}$	a.	0-6 mm Hg
_____	12.	RVSP	b.	4-12 mm Hg
_____	13.	RVDP	c.	8-15 mm Hg
_____	14.	PASP	d.	10-15 mm Hg
_____	15.	PADP	e.	15-25 mm Hg
_____	16.	PAMP	f.	60-80 mm Hg
_____	17.	PAWP	g.	70-95 mm Hg
_____	18.	LAP	h.	100-130 mm Hg
_____	19.	LVSP	i.	100-140 mm Hg
_____	20.	LVDP		
_____	21.	AOS		
_____	22.	AOD		
_____	23.	AOMEAN		

Match the following heart and pulmonary pressure waveforms:

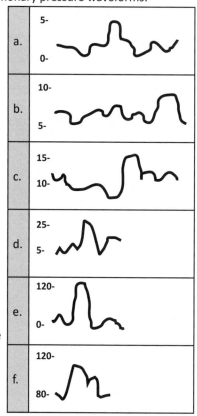

24. _____ Right atrium

25. _____ Right ventricle

26. _____ Left ventricle

27. _____ Pulmonary artery

28. _____ Pulmonary wedge

29. _____ Aorta

Match the following parameters with the appropriate description

	Parameter		Normal Range
____	30. a wave	a.	Bulging of A-V valve
____	31. c wave	b.	Passive atrial emptying
____	32. v wave	c.	Venous inflow into atria with closed A-V valves
____	33. x descent	d.	Atrial systole
____	34. y descent	e.	Atrial relaxation

35. Myocardial O_2 supply is determined by:
    a. Preload and afterload
    b. Heart rate and contracility
    c. CaO_2 and stroke volume
    d. Coronary blood flow and CaO_2

36. Coronary perfusion pressure is estimated clinically by:
    a. Aos - Coronary Venous Pressure
    b. AOD - Coronary Venous Pressure
    c. BPdia - PAWP
    d. BPdia - CVP

37. Arterial blood pressure equals:
    a. CO / BSA
    b. CO x SVR
    c. HR x SV
    d. CI / BSA

38. Cardiac output equals:
    a. CO / BSA
    b. CO / SVR
    c. HR x SV
    d. CI / BSA

39. Normal cardiac index equals:
    a. 2.5 – 4.2 L/min/m²
    b. 4-8 L/min/m²
    c. < 2.2 L/min/m²
    d. 60-80 mm Hg

40. The dicrotic notch of the arterial blood pressure waveform represents:
    a. Closure of the aortic semilunar valve
    b. Closure of the mitral valve
    c. Pressure rise due to blood entering the aorta
    d. Pressure fall due to blood entering the aorta

41. Ejection fraction equals:
    a. SV / HR
    b. SV / EDV
    c. SV – EDV
    d. SV x HR

42. LVSW equals:
    a. SV x HR x 0.0136
    b. SV / (BP – PAWP) x 0.0136
    c. SV x ($\overline{BP}$ – PAWP) x 0.0136
    d. SW x (BPsys) x 0.0136

43. Preload is defined as:
    a. Muscle fiber length at end-systole
    b. Muscle fiber length at end-diastole
    c. Filling pressure at end-systole
    d. Filling pressure at mid-diastole

44. What is the upper physiological limit of LVEDP for improved LV function?
    a. 6-10 mm Hg
    b. 4-12 mm Hg
    c. 15-18 mm Hg
    d. > 20 mm Hg

45. Preload is clinically measured by:
    a. CVP or PAWP
    b. RVEDV or LVEDV
    c. Both a or b
    d. Neither a nor b

46. Afterload is defined as:
    a. Total force causing ventricular ejection
    b. Total force opposing ventricular ejection
    c. Pressure the heart must develop for total ejection
    d. Pressure heart develops at end-diastole

47. The clinical measure of RV afterload is:
    a. PASP + PVR
    b. PADP + PVR
    c. PAMP – PVR
    d. CVP – PVR

48. The clinical measure of LV afterload is:
    a. BPsys + SVR
    b. BPdia + SVR
    c. $\overline{BP}$ – SVR
    d. PAWP – SVR

49. Contractility is defined as the:
    a. Ability to contract dependent on preload and afterload
    b. Chronotropic state of myocardium
    c. Inotropic state of myocardium
    d. Ability to return to preload state

50. LV contractility is proportional to:
    a. LVSV
    b. LVSVI
    c. LVSW
    d. LVSWI

51. Systemic vascular resistance is measured by:
    a. $[(\overline{BP} - CVP) / CO]$ x 80
    b. $[(\overline{BP} - PAWP) / CO]$ x 80
    c. $[(\overline{BP} - CVP) \times CO]$ x 80
    d. $[(\overline{BP} - PAWP) \times CO]$ x 80

52. Normal SVR equals:
    a. 20-200 dynes•sec•cm^{-5}
    b. 100-250 dynes•sec•cm^{-5}
    c. 800-1600 dynes•sec•cm-$^{-5}$
    d. 1000-2000 dynes•sec•cm^{-5}

53. SVR is increased by:
    a. Vasoconstriction
    b. Vasodilation
    c. Increased vessel distensibility
    d. None of the above

54. Pulmonary vascular resistance is measured by:
    a. $[(PAWP - PAMP) / CO]$ x 80
    b. $[(PADP-PAWP) / CO]$ x 80
    c. $[(PASP - PADP) \times CO]$ x 80
    d. $[(PAMP - PAWP) / CO]$ x 80

55. Normal PVR equals:
    a. 20-200 dynes•sec•cm^{-5}
    b. 60-100 dynes•sec•cm^{-5}
    c. 800-1600 dynes•sec•cm-$^{-5}$
    d. 1000-2000 dynes•sec•cm^{-5}

1. A 32-year-old man is preparing to run a marathon. Summarize what is likely to occur in terms of oxygen supply and demand during the marathon.

2. Explain physiologically what the difference is between systole and diastole in the context of arterial blood pressure. Be sure to include details about what is happening during each.

3. Fill in the table:

	Brief Definition (in your own words)	Clinical Measures	Factors that ↑	Factors that ↓
Preload				
Afterload				
Contractility				

4. A patient who makes his living as a sherpa in very high altitudes has polycythemia.
    a. Why does the sherpa most likely have polycythemia?

    b. What effect does the polycythemia have on preload, afterload, and contractility? Explain your answer.

5. A patient has an increase is myocardial oxygen demand and a normal myocardial oxygen supply. What will happen to the myocardial oxygen reserve in this case? Why is this scenario unlikely to occur in the absence of disease?

Match the following:

Parameter		Normal Range	
_____	1. O_2 supply	a.	SaO_2
_____	2. O_2 demand	b.	$S\bar{v}O_2$
_____	3. O_2 reserve	c.	$\dot{V}O_2$

4. Which of the following is true of SaO_2 monitoring?
   a. It is an early indicator of hypoxemia
   b. It adequately assesses ventilatory support
   c. It adequately assesses the effectiveness of respiratory interventions
   d. All of the above are true

5. A patient is on a nonrebreathing oxygen mask at 12 L/min and pulse oximetry (SpO_2) after being transported by EMS, who rescued the patient from a house fire. The SpO_2 is currently reading 100%. Which of the following is most appropriate?
   a. Maintain the nonrebreather as the SpO_2 is potentially inaccurate
   b. Decrease the flow on the nonrebreather to wean oxygen
   c. Immediately intubate the patient and place on mechanical ventilation
   d. Switch patient to a 50% venti mask to decrease delivered oxygen while increasing delivered flow

6. A measured $S\bar{v}O_2$ value of 44% is noted. Which of the following are potential causes of the value?
   1. Acute MI
   2. Septic Shock
   3. Anxiety causes by suctioning, pain, etc.
   4. Hypothermia
   5. Fever

   a. 1, 2, and 5
   b. 1, 3, and 5
   c. 2, 3, and 5
   d. 2, 4, and 5

7. The pulse rate of the pulse oximeter is noted to be much lower than that of the heart rate monitor. What should the Respiratory Therapist do next?
   a. Draw an Arterial Blood Gas and correlate values
   b. Call a *Code Blue* and begin high quality chest compressions
   c. Warm the monitoring site and replace sensor
   d. Move the oximeter probe site and recheck

8. A patient is in the ICU, currently being monitored with EKG leads, a non-invasive blood pressure cuff on the left arm, and a central line in the right subclavian vein. Which of the following is the most appropriate initial placement of a pulse oximeter probe?
   a. Left nare
   b. Left pointer finger
   c. Right ring finger
   d. Right ear lobe

9. Oxygen supply is best represented by:
   a. $\dot{V}O_2$
   b. $S\bar{v}O_2$
   c. $C\bar{v}O_2$
   d. SaO_2

Answer the following as True (T) or False (F)

_____ 10. SaO_2 refers to invasive monitoring of oxygenation

_____ 11. SpO_2 refers to the noninvasive monitoring of oxygenation, also called pulse oximetry

_____ 12. The normal acceptable clinical range for both SaO_2 and SpO_2 is 80-100%

_____ 13. SpO_2 is a reliable indicator of SaO_2 in the presence of dysfunctional hemoglobins

_____ 14. $S\bar{v}O_2$ monitoring is the intermittent or continuous monitoring of mixed venous blood

_____ 15. $S\bar{v}O_2$ is a measure of the amount of O_2 consumed by body tissues

_____ 16. $SvO_2 = SaO_2 - Sa - \bar{v}O_2$

_____ 17. $S\bar{v}O_2$ indicates whether oxygen supply is meeting oxygen demand

_____ 18. Mixed venous blood is present in the RA, RV, and pulmonary arteries

_____ 19. Normal SvO_2 is > 75%

_____ 20. An $S\bar{V}O_2 < 50\%$ reflects the O_2 reserve is used up

_____ 21. An $S\bar{V}O_2 > 80\%$ suggests oxygen supply is greater than oxygen demand

_____ 22. When the $S\bar{V}O_2$ is normal, the cardiovascular status is always normal

For each of the following physiological causes, indicate whether it results in an increased SvO_2 (↑) or a decreased SvO_2 (↓).

23. _____ Increased arterial O_2 supply

24. _____ Increased tissue demand

25. _____ Right-to-Left shunt

26. _____ Decreased arterial O_2 supply

27. _____ Left-to-Right shunt

28. _____ Decreased tissue demand

Chapter 3
Test Questions

1. $S\bar{v}O_2$ equals:
   a. $SaO_2 + S\bar{v}O_2$
   b. $SaO_2 - Sa\text{-}\bar{v}O_2$
   c. $SaO_2 - \dot{V}O_2$
   d. $SaO_2 / \dot{V}O_2$

2. Normal acceptable clinical range of SaO_2 is:
   a. > 75%
   b. > 85%
   c. > 90%
   d. > 95%

3. SpO_2 may be a poor indicator of SaO_2:
   a. In the absence of dysfunctional hemoglobin
   b. In the presence of dysfunctional hemoglobin
   c. SpO_2 is always a poor indicator of SaO_2
   d. Never: SpO_2 always accurately indicates SaO_2

4. The only consistent clinical correlate of $S\bar{v}O_2$ is:
   a. SaO_2
   b. $S\bar{v}O_2$
   c. SpO_2
   d. O_2ER

5. $S\bar{v}O2$ changes often _____ significant hemodynamic changes:
   a. Precede
   b. Come after
   c. Accompany
   d. Don't relate to

6. Normal $S\bar{v}O_2$ range equals:
   a. 5 – 10%
   b. 40 – 60%
   c. 60 – 80%
   d. 80 – 100%

7. A decrease in $S\bar{v}O_2$ of $\geq$ 10% for $\geq$ 3 minutes is:
   a. Clinically insignificant
   b. Impending deterioration
   c. The beginning of anaerobic metabolism
   d. Indicative of insufficient tissue O_2

8. The most common cause of a decreased $S\bar{v}O_2$ is:
   a. Decreased CO
   b. Decreased CaO_2
   c. Increased CO
   d. Increased CaO_2

9. A pulse volume amplitude of 4 equals a(n) _____ pulse:
   a. Absent
   b. Diminished
   c. Normal
   d. Bounding

10. *Pulsus paradoxicus* is best defined as:
    a. Regular alternation of weak and strong pulses
    b. Regular alternation of pulse with respiration
    c. Decreased pulse volume with inspiration and increased with expiration
    d. Decreased pulse volume with expiration and increased with inspiration

Chapter 3
Critical Thinking Questions

1. Answer the following questions about $S\bar{v}O_2$:

   a. Briefly define $S\bar{v}O_2$.

   b. At what point is blood considered mixed?

   c. How are these samples obtained?

2. What type of shunt results in an increased $S\bar{v}O_2$? Explain the physiology behind why this results in an increase.

1. A Central Line obtains the following type of samples:
    a. Arterial
    b. Venous
    c. Mixed Arterial
    d. Mixed Venous

2. An Arterial Line (A-Line) obtains the following type of samples:
    a. Arterial
    b. Venous
    c. Mixed Arterial
    d. Mixed Venous

3. The proximal port of a Pulmonary Artery Line obtains the following type of samples:
    a. Arterial
    b. Venous
    c. Mixed Arterial
    d. Mixed Venous

4. The distal port of a Pulmonary Artery Line obtains the following type of samples:
    a. Arterial
    b. Venous
    c. Mixed Arterial
    d. Mixed Venous

5. Which of the following is FALSE when obtaining samples from invasive lines:
    a. Only the amount necessary should be obtained
    b. Samples from lines should not be used for blood cultures
    c. As many samples as possible should be drawn simultaneously
    d. Drawing from a left atrium line is preferable to prevent potential embolization

Answer the following as True (T) or False (F)

_____ 1. Palpation of an arterial pulse can reveal rate, rhythm, volume, and systolic blood pressure

_____ 2. *Pulsus alternans* is the regular alternation of weak and strong pulses

_____ 3. *Pulsus paradoxicus* is noted when the volume of the pulse increases on inspiration

_____ 4. The American Heart Association (AHA) recommends recording three pressures when auscultating blood pressure

_____ 5. The two indicators for an intra-arterial catheter are blood pressure monitoring and arterial blood gas sampling

Match the following:

Equipment		Purpose
_____ 6.	Amplifier	a. Holding device
_____ 7.	Flush device	b. Display device
_____ 8.	Manifold	c. Prevent clotting
_____ 9.	Monitor	d. Converts mechanical to electrical energy
_____ 10.	Transducer	e. An electrical device which amplifies an electrical signal

11. Balancing the transducer to <u>atmopsheric pressure</u> is referred to as:
    a. Calibration
    b. Zeroing
    c. Reverse-calibration
    d. Settling

12. Balancing the transducer to <u>a known pressure</u> is referred to as:
    a. Calibration
    b. Zeroing
    c. Reverse-calibration
    d. Settling

13. A-line pressure bags should be kept at (mm Hg):
    a. 15
    b. 120
    c. 250
    d. 300

14. When performing a modified Allen's test, adequate circulation will return color within how many seconds?
    a. 7 or less
    b. 10 or less
    c. 15 or less
    d. 30 or less

15. If the distal pulse becomes absent after placement of an arterial line:
    a. An embolectomy should be performed
    b. The catheter should be removed
    c. The catheter should be secured, and the observation documented
    d. The catheter should be flushed with copious amounts of heparin

16. When flushing an arterial line, the Respiratory Therapist should:
    a. Not aspirate the line before flushing
    b. Ensure flushing is completed even if blood return is not obtained
    c. Perform flushing quickly and forcefully
    d. Perform flushing slowly with small volumes

17. A primary source of arterial line infections is:
    a. The stopcock
    b. Insertion of the catheter
    c. The clinician's hands
    d. What is infused

18. What arterial pressure increases in distal vessels?
    a. BPsys
    b. BPdia
    c. $\overline{BP}$
    d. AOD

19. Of the following, which is the preferred arterial site for placement of an intra-arterial catheter?
    a. Axillary
    b. Dorsalis Pedis
    c. Radial
    d. Brachial

Match the following:

	Arterial Waveform Variation		Description
_____	20.	Pulsus alternans	a. Strong, bounding pulse
_____	21.	Pulsus biferiens	b. Weak pulse
_____	22.	Pulsus paradoxicus	c. Two systolic peaks
_____	23.	Pulsus parva	d. Every other beat is weaker
_____	24.	Pulsus bigeminus	e. Every other beat is larger
_____	25.	Pulsus Corrigans	f. Decreased BPsys during inspiration

Chapter 5
Test Questions

Match the following:

		Arterial Waveform Variation		Description
_____	1.	BPsys	a.	CO x SVR
_____	2.	BPdia	b.	LV systolic pressure
_____	3.	$\overline{BP}$	c.	SV and arterial compliance
_____	4.	PP	d.	Runoff and aortic elasticity

5. The arterial pressure waveform reflects changes in the:
   a. RV and LV
   b. LV and SVR
   c. RV and LA
   d. LV and PAWP

6. Which arterial line pressure increases in distal vessels?
   a. BPsys
   b. BPdia
   c. $\overline{BP}$
   d. Brachial

7. Intra-arterial Catheters (A-Lines) are indicated for which of the following?
   1. ACLS drug administration
   2. Fluid maintenance
   3. Monitoring of blood pressure when unstable
   4. Arterial blood gas sampling
   5. Monitoring of blood pressure in assessing therapeutic interventions

   a. 1, 2, and 4
   b. 1, 3, and 5
   c. 3, 4, and 5
   d. 1, 2, 3, 4, and 5

8. Which of the following is true regarding zeroing and calibrating an A-Line?
   a. The transducer should be calibrated to a known pressure using a mercury manometer
   b. The patient should be placed in a supine or nearly-supine position
   c. The monitoring system should generally be zeroed before warming it up
   d. Zeroing is the process of manually setting the zero value against a known manufacturer pressure

Match the following:

	Arterial Waveform Variation		Description
_____	9.	Pulsus alternans	a. Strong, bounding pulse
_____	10.	Pulsus biferiens	b. Two systolic peaks
_____	11.	Pulsus bigeminus	c. Weak pulse
_____	12.	Pulsus corrigans	d. Every other beat is larger
_____	13.	Pulsus paradoxicus	e. Every other beat is weaker
_____	14.	Pulsus prava	f. Decreased BPsys during inspiration

15. RVEDP equals:
    a. RV emptying pressure
    b. RV filling pressure
    c. RV mean pressure
    d. RV peak pressure

16. The phlebostatic axis is located where?
    a. Approximately at the level of the right ventricle
    b. Midaxillary at 5th intercostal space
    c. Both A and B are correct
    d. Niether A nor B are correct

17. A blood pressure from an indwelling arterial catheter is measured at 110/88. Calculate the mean arterial pressure (in mm Hg).
    a. 66
    b. 99
    c. 95
    d. 103

18. When recording a blood pressure, you are actually recording:
    a. Contraction and then relaxation of the ventricles
    b. Normal physiologic vasospasm and relaxation of brachial artery
    c. Pulmonary artery response to oxygen content
    d. Relaxation and then contraction of the ventricles

19. Using a blood pressure cuff that is too small or too loose may result in:
    a. A falsely high diastolic reading with a normal systolic reading
    b. A falsely low blood pressure
    c. A falsely low diastolic reading with a normal systolic reading
    d. A falsely high blood pressure

20. Of the following, which is the preferred arterial site for placement of an intra-arterial catheter?
    a. Femoral
    b. Axillary
    c. Radial
    d. Brachial

21. A radial A-line has been in place for several hours. The Respiratory Therapist notices that the waveform is dampened on the monitor. Which of the following are potential causes of this?
    1. Loose connection
    2. Catheter tip against vessel wall
    3. Electrical interference
    4. Blood clot on catheter tip
    5. Patient movement

    a. 1, 2, and 4
    b. 1, 3, and 5
    c. 3, 4, and 5
    d. 1, 2, 3, 4, and 5

22. A blood pressure from a femoral arterial blood gas is measured at 90/50. Calculate the mean arterial pressure (in mm Hg).
    a. 63
    b. 70
    c. 77
    d. 40

1. A left femoral A-Line was placed on a critical care patient 1 day ago. The doppler pulse in the left foot is noted to be absent. The patient is not hemodynamically stable. Explain what steps should occur next.

2. List the basic steps involved in drawing an arterial sample from a typical A-line. For each step list any relevant potential hazards as well as at least one way to prevent each hazard.

3. A 52-year-old male has an arterial line placed in the right radial artery. The waveform is noted to slowly rise through the anacrotic limb, followed by a partially diminished dicrotic notch. Invasive blood pressure is 90/72.

a. What is the systolic pressure?
    Is this normal, abnormally low, or abnormally high?

b. What is the diastolic pressure?
    Is this normal, abnormally low, or abnormally high?

c. What is the pulse pressure?
    Is this normal, abnormally low, or abnormally high?

d. What is the mean blood pressure?
    Is this normal, abnormally low, or abnormally high?

e. Based on the clinical presentation, what pathological condition is most supported? Give evidence (what features support your potential diagnosis?).

4. An 18-year-old female has been hospitalized for massive trauma following a rollover motor vehicle crash with prolonged extrication. She has an arterial line placed in the right radial artery. In trying to draw a sample, the Respiratory Therapist observes that no blood will draw up when trying to aspirate the line. List the potential causes, and then give possible interventions for each cause.

1. The Central Venous Pressure (CVP) is <u>not</u> equal to the pressure in the:
   a. Superior vena cava
   b. Distal inferior vena cava
   c. Right atrium
   d. Proximal inferior vena cava

2. The indications for monitoring via a Central line (CVP) include:
   a. Assessment of right heart function
   b. Assessment of left heart function
   c. Assessment of intravascular volume status
   d. All of the above

3. Central Venous Pressures are often accurate in the presence of:
   a. Left-to-right shunt
   b. Cardiomyopathy
   c. Tricuspid insufficiency
   d. Left heart dysfunction

4. Which of the following equations most accurately represents venous return to the heart?
   a. BP - CVP
   b. BP + CVP
   c. $\overline{BP}$ - CVP
   d. $\overline{\overline{BP}}$ + CVP

5. Insertion sites for a central line include all of the following, <u>except</u>:
   a. Superior vena cava
   b. Internal jugular vein
   c. Subclavian vein
   d. Femoral vein

6. Once placed, central vein catheter position may be confirmed by:
   a. Catheter length
   b. Measurement of PaO_2
   c. Pressure waveform
   d. X-ray

Answer the following as True (T) or False (F)

_____ 7. CVP monitoring equipment is the same as for an A-line, but uses a different catheter

_____ 8. The cutdown insertion technique is always the first choice in placing a central line

_____ 9. When drawing a blood sample from a jugular or subclavian CVP line, the patient should be as flat as possible

_____ 10. If a drug is being infused, always use it to flush after withdrawing a blood sample

_____ 11. When estimating CVP by neck veins the patient should be at a semi-Fowlers (45°) angle

_____ 12. When measuring CVP by the water manometer technique, the patient should be as level (flat) as possible

_____ 13. The phlebostatic axis is at the approximate level of the left atrium

_____ 14. The phlebostatic axis is the midaxillary point on the lateral chest in the 5th intercostal space

_____ 15. When measuring CVP by the water manometer technique, always remove the patient from the ventilator and/or PEEP

_____ 16. Serial trend measurements are not as clinically significant as individual readings

_____ 17. When measuring CVP using the transducer monitoring technique, the transducer levels should be + 5 cm above the phlebostatic axis

_____ 18. Normal CVP is 0-8 mm Hg

For each of the following, indicate whether it results in an increased CVP (↑) or a decreased CVP (↓).

19. _____ Spontaneous inspiration

20. _____ Spontaneous exhalation

21. _____ Positive pressure inspiration

22. _____ Fluid overload

23. _____ Hypovolemia

Match the following:

Waveform Part		Description
_____	1. a wave	a. Bulging of tricuspid valve into right atrium
_____	2. c wave	b. Right atrial contraction
_____	3. v wave	c. Right atrial relaxation
_____	4. x descent	d. Right atrial emptying

5. CVP measurements:
   a. Should be expressed in cm H_2O
   b. Should be made at end-inspiration
   c. Should include both systolic and diastolic pressures
   d. Should identify trends as more important than absolute values

6. Central Venous Pressure usually increases during:
   a. Spontaeous exhalation
   b. Spontaneous inspiration
   c. Cardiac arrest
   d. Positive pressure exhalation

7. Central Venous Pressure correlates most closely with:
   a. Right atrial pressure
   b. Left atrial pressure
   c. Pulmonary veins
   d. Peripheral venules

8. Which of the following result in an increased central venous pressure?
   1. Cor pulmonale
   2. Pulmonary hypertension
   3. Cardiac tamponade
   4. Catheter tip in the right ventricle
   5. Hypovolemic shock

   a. 1, 2, 3, and 4
   b. 1, 2, 3, and 5
   c. 1, 2, 4, and 5
   d. 2, 3, 4, and 5

9. A central line transducer has been zeroed and calibrated and placed 2 cm above the phlebostatic point. The patient is positioned in supine position. The CVP displays as 6 mm Hg. What is the true CVP (mm Hg)?
    a. 2
    b. 6
    c. 8
    d. Unable to determine with information provided

10. A 17-year-old male arrives in the Emergency Department with multiple gunshot wounds to the torso. A central line is placed. What would be expected to be true of the CVP?
    a. It would be lower than normal
    b. It would be unaffected (normal)
    c. It would be higher than normal
    d. It is not measurable in this clinical situation

11. A 22-year-old female is in the Surgical Intensive Care Unit. She has a sub-clavian central line with levophed being infused. A blood sample needs to be drawn. Which of the following is true?
    a. The infusion should be temporarily paused and a sample drawn
    b. The infusion should be discontinued to facilitate blood draws
    c. The infusion should not be paused - the blood should be obtained by a peripheral IV or other source
    d. Central lines can never be used for blood draws

12. The CVP catheter tip should optimally sit:
    a. In the jugular vein
    b. In the right atrium
    c. In the pulmonary artery
    d. In the left atrium

Answer the following as True (T) or False (F)

_____ 13. The *a wave* in the CVP waveform represents right ventricular contraction

_____ 14. The Central Venous Pressure (CVP) waveform is identical to the right atrial waveform

_____ 15. When measuring CVP with a transducer, the patient should be at a 45° angle

Chapter 6
Critical Thinking Questions

1. A 30-year-old female who is in septic shock has been aggressively fluid resusictated. A central line has been placed to carefully monitor her fluid status. While turning the patient her EKG suddenly displays V-tach.

   a. What is likely causing this change in EKG?

   b. What steps should be taken to correct this arrhythmia?

2. An 88-year-old male arrives in the Emergency Department. The Respiratory Therapist observes obvious jugular venous distension.
   a. What does jugular venous distension (JVD) suggest diagnostically?

   b. The phlebostatic axis is estimated to be approximately 14 centimeters. What is the estimated CVP? Is this normal, low, or high?

1. Indications for pulmonary artery pressure monitoring include all of the following, except:
   a. Assess heart function
   b. Monitor PvO_2
   c. Assess pulmonary function
   d. Diagnose, manage, and treat certain diseases

Match the following:

		PA Catheter Ports		Description
_____	2.	Balloon inflation port	a.	To measure CO
_____	3.	Distal lumen port	b.	To measure CVP
_____	4.	Proximal lumen port	c.	To measure $S\bar{v}O_2$
_____	5.	Thermistor connector port	d.	To inflate balloon

Answer the following as True (T) or False (F)

_____ 6. Before insertion, the PA catheter balloon should be tested for leaks by filling with a fluid

_____ 7. Deflation of the balloon should be done with negative pressure to ensure complete deflation

_____ 8. The balloon should always be slightly overinflated to maintain the balloon's integrity

_____ 9. PA catheter insertion sites are the same as CVP insertion sites

_____ 10. During insertion, the balloon should be inflated only after traversing the pulmonic valve

_____ 11. Pressures and waveforms should be monitored as the catheter is advanced

_____ 12. During insertion, once the PA occlusion occurs and the balloon is deflated, the wedge waveform should remain

Match the following:

	PA Catheter Pressure		Description
_____	13.	$\overline{RAP}$	a. 0-6 mm Hg
_____	14.	PASP	b. 4-12 mm Hg
_____	15.	PADP	c. 8-15 mm Hg
_____	16.	PAWP	d. 15-25 mm Hg

17. To record a wedge (PAWP) pressure:
   a. The wedge pressure should always be obtained with less than manufacturer-recommended balloon volume
   b. The PAWP should be recorded during expiration
   c. A large volume syringe should be used
   d. The balloon should be inflated slowly

18. Verification of a true wedge includes:
   a. Upon balloon inflation the PA waveform flattens to an LA waveform
   b. PAWP > PADP
   c. A blood sample from the distal port will be poorly saturated with O_2
   d. Upon balloon deflation the PAWP waveform appears

Answer the following as True (T) or False (F)

_____ 19. Balloon rupture may be detected using a glass syringe

_____ 20. IV solutions, drugs, and blood products should only be infused via the proximal port

_____ 21. Proper tip placement is verified by continuous monitoring of the proximal port waveform

_____ 22. PAWP and waveform should be checked every 8 hours

_____ 23. When drawing a mixed venous blood sample, the balloon should be inflated to prevent contamination from capillary blood

For each of the following, indicate whether the parameter is Measured (M) or Derived (D)

24. _____ CO

25. _____ CI

26. _____ CVP

27. _____ $C\bar{v}O_2$

28. _____ HR

29. _____ LV function curve

30. _____ PAMP

31. _____ PAWP

32. _____ $P\bar{v}CO_2$

33. _____ $S\bar{v}O_2$

34. _____ PVR

35. _____ SV

36. The primary cause of a decreased PAP is:
    a. L-R shunt
    b. Increased PVR
    c. Hypovolemia
    d. Left ventricular failure

37. The primary cause of a decreased PAWP is:
    a. Cardiac tamponade
    b. Hypovolemia
    c. Hypervolemia
    d. Pneumothorax

38. The pulmonary artery wedge pressure at which acute pulmonary edema occurs is approximately (mm Hg):
    a. 12
    b. 18
    c. 25
    d. 30

39. Which of the following represents the normal relationship between pulmonary artery wedge pressure and left ventricular end diastolic pressure?
    a. PAWP ≠ LVEDP
    b. PAWP ≈ LVEDP
    c. PAWP < LVEDP
    d. PAWP > LVEDP

40. The normal PADP – PAWP gradient is (mm Hg):
    a. 0
    b. 0-6
    c. 5-10
    d. > 10

41. The PAP waveform is similar to, but smaller than, the:
    a. A-line pressure waveform
    b. CVP waveform
    c. RV pressure waveform
    d. LV pressure waveform

42. The PAWP waveform is least similar to the:
    a. CVP waveform
    b. RAP waveform
    c. LAP waveform
    d. PAP waveform

For each of the following, indicate whether the Pulmonary Artery Baseline Pressure (PAP) will Increase (I) or Decrease (D)

43. _____ Spontaenous inspiration

44. _____ Spontaneous exhalation

45. _____ Positive pressure ventilation: inspiration

46. _____ Positive pressure ventilation: exhalation

47. When a PAP (mm Hg) suddenly changes from 20/0 to 20/10, the following has most likely occurred:
   a. Increased PVR
   b. Decreased PVR
   c. The catheter tip has slipped into the right ventricle
   d. The catheter tip has spontaneously wedged

48. All pressure reading of PASP, PAMP, PADP, and PAWP should be taken:
   a. During inspiration
   b. During exhalation
   c. At end-inspiration
   d. At end-exhalation

49. Inaccurate PAP and PAWP usually occur when the patient's head-up position exceeds:
   a. 10°
   b. 20°
   c. 30°
   d. 45°

For each of the following, indicate the appropriate Lung Zone (1, 2, or 3)

50. _____ Majority of the lung

51. _____ Uppermost portion of the lung

52. _____ Vascular channel is continually closed

53. _____ Vascular channel closes during exhalation

54. _____ PAWP ≠ LAP

55. _____ Lung zone that decreases with PEEP

56. _____ PA > Pa > Pv

57. _____ Pa > PA > Pv

58. _____ Pa > Pv > PA

59. Postiive pressure during inspiration may cause all of the following, except:
    a. Decreased CO
    b. Increased PAWP
    c. Increased zone 1 and zone 2
    d. Decreased PEEP

Answer the following as True (T) or False (F)

_____ 60. PEEP often exaggerates the cardiovascular effects of positive pressure ventilation

_____ 61. The cardiovascular effects of positive pressure ventilation decrease as lung compliance decreases

_____ 62. Cardiovascular effects of positive presure ventilation are most directly proportional to the increased PIT

_____ 63. Measured PAWP is almost always an overestimation of true PAWP when on postiive pressure ventilation and PEEP

_____ 64. As PEEP levels are increased, zones 1 and 2 also increase

_____ 65. When PAWP increases by at least half of the added PEEP, then the catheter tip is likely in zone 3

_____ 66. Because of the cardiovascular effects, the patient is best removed from positive pressure ventilation during the recording of PAWP

67. Clinical indications of balloon rupture include all the following except:
    a. Failure to wedge
    b. Resistance during inflation
    c. Blood in balloon lumen
    d. PA waveform persists after inflation

68. A proper step to take in the event of a suspected balloon rupture is:
    a. Attempt to inflate with air at least 3 times to ensure rupture
    b. Ensure no further wedge attempts after the one confirmation attempt
    c. Remove catheter immediately
    d. Never use CO_2 to test for the rupture

Answer the following as True (T) or False (F)

_____ 69. When aspiration fails to produce a blood return and a blood clot is suspected, the system should immediately be flushed to attempt to remove the clot

_____ 70. Flushing should always be done in the wedge position

_____ 71. Clinical evidence of a ruptured artery may include aspiration if air throughout the distal lumen and hemoptysis

_____ 72. Massive hemoptysis is evidenced by a quantity of blood greater than 15 mL

_____ 73. Prolonged wedging beyond 15 seconds may result in pulmonary ischemia

_____ 74. Pulmonary artery catheters should be removed after 7 days

Answer the following as True (T) or False (F)

_____ 1. Pulmonary artery pressure monitoring can assess both right and left heart function

_____ 2. PA catheter insertion sites are the same as CVP insertion

_____ 3. PA catheter balloons should always be test-inflated with fluid and not air

_____ 4. During insertion, once the PA occlusion position is reached, the balloon must be immediately deflated

_____ 5. Normal PADP is 15-25 mm hg

_____ 6. Balloon inflation should stop when the PA waveform changes to the PAWP waveform

_____ 7. Upon balloon inflation, the PA waveform should flatten to an LA waveform

_____ 8. Wedge time should always be less than 10 seconds

9. Measurements obtained witha PA line include all of the following, except:
   a. $C\bar{v}O_2$
   b. PVR
   c. SWI
   d. SVRI

10. PVR is proportional to:
   a. PASP - PADP gradient
   b. PAMP - PADP gradient
   c. PADP - PAWP gradient
   d. PAMP - PAWP gradient

11. The major cause for decreased PAP is
   a. Hypovolemia
   b. Hypervolemia
   c. Sepsis
   d. Right heart failure

12. The main cause for a decreased PAWP is:
    a. Hypovolemia
    b. Hypervolemia
    c. Sepsis
    d. Right heart failure

13. Acute pulmonary edema occurs when:
    a. PADP > 30 mm Hg
    b. PAMP > 30 mm Hg
    c. PAWP > 30 mm Hg
    d. PASP > 30 mm Hg

14. PADP < PAWP equals:
    a. 0-6 mmHg
    b. Pulmonary embolism
    c. Backwards flow
    d. Overwedged catheter tip

15. During positive pressure inspiration, the PA waveform baseline pressure:
    a. Increases
    b. Decreases
    c. Stays the same
    d. No longer reflects true pressure

16. During positive pressure inspiration, the PAWP waveform baseline pressure:
    a. Increases
    b. Decreases
    c. Stays the same
    d. No longer reflects true pressure

17. During PAP measuring, body positition should be:
    a. Head up 0-20°
    b. Head up > 20°
    c. Head up 0-45°
    d. Head up 45°

18. The PA catheter tip should remain in lung zone:
    a. 1
    b. 2
    c. 3
    d. 2 and 3

19. During labored spontaneous breathing, hemodynamic parameters:
    a. Are minimally affected
    b. Mimic positive pressure breaths
    c. Are reversed from normal spontaneous breathing
    d. None of the above

20. Cardiovascular effects of positive pressure ventilation are directly proportional to:
    a. PIC
    b. PIP
    c. PIT
    d. PIV

21. PEEP causes:
    a. Increased lung zones 1 and 2
    b. Decreased lung zones 1 and 2
    c. Increased lung zones 2 and 3
    d. Decreased lung zones 2 and 3

1. Answer the following questions regarding inflating the balloon into a wedge position with the Pulmonary Artery Cathter

    a. Explain the process of wedging - what is actually happening?

    b. What is being less directly measured when wedging?

    c. The wedge maneuver is a short maneuver. What would happen if the balloon were left in wedge position (with balloon inflated)?

2. Why are Pulmonary Artery Catheters not placed in more critical care patients? The information seems like it could be beneficial for anyone who is not hemodnyamically stable.

3. A patient has had a Pulmonary Artery Catheter (PA Catheter) placed. The following values (mm Hg) are obtained:

RAP	5
RVSP	20
RVEDP	5
PAP	30/20
PAMP	23
PAOP (PCWP)	10

   a. Interpret each value as normal or abnormal (high, low).

   b. This patient is now intubated and placed on a positive pressure ventilator. The following settings are used:

Mode	Pressure Assist/Control
Inspiratory Pressure	16 cm H₂O
PEEP	5 cm H₂O
Set Rate	15 breaths/min
Inspiratory Time	0.9 seconds
Oxygen %	50%

   What effects will these settings have on the hemodynamic parameters above? Be specific.

Match the following:

		Parameter		Description
_____	1.	Cardiac Index	a.	SV / EDV
_____	2.	Cardiac output	b.	$\dfrac{\overline{PAP} - PAWP \times 80}{CO}$
_____	3.	Ejection fraction	c.	CO / BSA
_____	4.	Stroke volume	d.	SV x Vpress
_____	5.	Stroke work	e.	CO / HR
_____	6.	Systemic vascular resistance	f.	$\dfrac{\overline{BP} - CVP \times 80}{CO}$
_____	7.	Pulmonary vascular resistance	g.	SV x HR

8. The most commonly used bedside determination of cardiac output is:
   a. Fick method
   b. Angigography method
   c. Indicator (dye) dilution
   d. Thermodilution method

9. During the thermodilution method, the PA catheter tip should be in:
   a. Zone 1
   b. Zone 2
   c. Zone 3
   d. Any zone is acceptable

10. When a patient is receiving mechanical ventilation, the thermodilution injectate should be injected:
   a. During inspiration
   b. At end-inspiration
   c. During exhalation
   d. At end-exhalation

1. A cardiac index of 1.6 L/min/m² indicates:
   a. Hyperperfusion
   b. Shock
   c. Normal cardiac output, adjusted to body size
   d. This value is not possible

2. A 23-year-old male with a complex medical history has a measured ejection fraction of 55%. The Respiratory Therapist would interpret this as:
   a. Serious ventricular dysfunction
   b. Profound ventricular dysfunction
   c. Normal ejection fraction
   d. Hyperperfusing

3. When measuring cardiac output of a patient on a positive pressure ventilator, injection should occur:
   a. At the start of inspiration
   b. At the start of exhalation
   c. End-inspiration
   d. End-exhalation

4. Of the following which are likely to cause a decrease in cardiac output?
   1. Acute myocardial infarction
   2. Early septic shock
   3. Late septic shock
   4. Coagulopathy

   a. 1, 2, and 3
   b. 1, 2, and 4
   c. 1, 3, and 4
   d. 2, 3, and 4

5. The pulmonary artery catheter tip is in the right ventricle. This is most likely to result in:
   a. Cardiac output value lower than expected
   b. Irregular upslope of CO curve
   c. Cardiac output value higher than expected
   d. Irregular downslope of CO curve

1. In your own words, explain what cardiac output is. Include the consequences of having too low and too high a cardiac output.

2. What is cardiac index? Why is it important to consider cardiac index in assessing a patient's hemodynamic status?

1. The purpose of the intraortic balloon pump is to increase oxygen supply to the myocardium during _____ and to decrease oxygen demand to the myocardium during _____:
   a. Diastole, Diastole
   b. Diastole, Systole
   c. Systole, Diastole
   d. Systole, Systole

2. The intraaortic balloon inflates during _____ and deflates during _____.
   a. Diastole, Systole
   b. Systole, Diastole
   c. Asystole, Diastole
   d. Systole, Asystole

3. Inflation of the IABP is also known as:
   a. Right ventricular augmentation
   b. Afterload reduction
   c. Diastolic augmentation
   d. Cardiac fortitude

4. Deflation of the IABP is also known as:
   a. Right ventricular augmentation
   b. Afterload reduction
   c. Diastolic augmentation
   d. Cardiac fortitude

5. A 28-year-old male has an IABP inserted, running at a beat ratio of 1:2. The patient goes into cardiac arrest. Which is the most likely to occur?
   a. Balloon deflates prematurely
   b. Monitor reads high systolic and low diastolic pressures
   c. Apperance of blood in the catheter
   d. Loss of cardiac signal

6. Which of the following would not be an expected hemodynamic change after initiation of the IABP?
   a. Increase in systolic pressure
   b. Increase in diastolic pressures
   c. Increase in cardiac output
   d. Decrease in heart rate

Answer the following as True (T) or False (F)

_____ 7. Balloon pumping is most effective with a heart rate of 80-120 beats/minute

_____ 8. Balloon pumping should be discontinued if tachycardia (rate > 120 bpm) occurs

_____ 9. Balloon pumping should be discontinued during cardiac arrest

_____ 10. Discontinuation criteria for the IABP includes a HR < 110 bpm; CI > 2.0; and $\overline{BP}$ > 70 mm Hg

1. The purpose of the IABP is to:
   a. Increase oxygen supply to the heart during diastole
   b. Decrease oxygen supply to the heart during diastole
   c. Increase oxygen supply to the heart during systole
   d. Decrease oxygen supply to the heart during systole

2. Diastolic augmentation results from:
   a. Inflation of the balloon
   b. Deflation of the balloon
   c. Systemic unloading
   d. Decreased systolic ejection time

3. Discontinuation criteria for the IABP includes all of the following, <u>except</u>:
   a. HR > 110 bpm
   b. $\overline{BP}$ > 70 mm Hg
   c. PAWP < 18 mm Hg
   d. CI > 2.0 L/min/m^2

4. A patient has an IABP inserted, running at a beat ratio of 1:2. The EKG is displaying Premature Ventricular Contractions (PVCs). What effect could this have on the IABP?
   a. Balloon deflates prematurely
   b. Monitor reads high systolic and low diastolic pressures
   c. Apperance of blood in the catheter
   d. Loss of cardiac signal

5. Goals of the IABP include:
   1. Decrease cytokine release
   2. Improve myocardial oxygenation
   3. Increase cardiac output
   4. Reduce left ventricular workload

   a. 1, 2, and 3
   b. 1, 2, and 4
   c. 1, 3, and 4
   d. 2, 3, and 4

6. Which of the following patients would be most appropriate for placement of an intraaortic balloon pump?
   a. A patient who just had a cardiopulmonary bypass
   b. A patient with a pulmonary embolism
   c. Prophylaxsis for a patient in a hypertensive crisis
   d. Emergent placement during cardiac arrest

7. Which of the following is true of IABP catheter placement?
   a. Catheter is inserted via a femoral artery and advanced into the right atrium
   b. Catheter is inserted via a brachial artery and advanced just beyond the first bifurcation of the pulmonary artery
   c. Catheter is inserted via a femoral artery and advanced into the descending aorta
   d. Catheter is inserted via a subclavian vein and advanced into the descending aorta

1. Explain in your own words how an intraortic balloon pump works.

2. The catheter is placed for the IABP in the most common vessel on the right side. The distal pulse is noted to be moderately diminished (from a classification of 2/4 to 1/4). What steps could have been taken to try to avoid this?

3. The IABP is not like other hemodynamic tools discussed in the pocket guide. It is a therapeutic device, and is usually weaned before being discontinued.
   a. How is the device weaned (there are 3 primary methods)?

   b. At what point would a patient on an IABP start to be weaned (give some specific criteria)?

Answer the following as True (T) or False (F)

_____ 1. In ARDS, an increased PVR does not occur until greater than 50% of the vascular bed is destroyed or obstructed

_____ 2. A chronic RV hypertrophy can produce a PASP of 70-90 mm Hg

_____ 3. PAWP is normal in ARDS and increased in cardiogenic pulmonary edema

_____ 4. Cardiac failure is synonymous with right heart failure (RHF), left heart failure (LHF), and congestive heart failure (CHF)

_____ 5. Right heart failure is called *Cor pulmonale* if due to lung disease

Match the following:

Failure Type	Most Commonly Results In:
Left heart failure	
_____ 6. Forward Failure	a. Cardiogenic shock
_____ 7. Backward Failure	b. Decreased pulmonary perfusion
Right heart failure	c. Pulmonary congestion
_____ 8. Forward Failure	d. Venous congestion
_____ 9. Backward Failure	

Answer the following as True (T) or False (F)

_____ 10. LHF is the most common cause of RHF

_____ 11. The common hemodynamic presentation of backward RHF is ↓ CVP

_____ 12. In cardiac tamponade, a diastolic pressure plateau is when: RAP = RVEDP = PAD = PAWP = LAP = LVEDP

_____ 13. The most common characteristic of cardiac myopathy is a decreased SV

_____ 14. A high PAWP in a COPD patient is likely the result of an enlarged lung zone 3

15. The three most common clinical manifestation of backward RHF are:
    a. Dyspnea, cough, orthopnea
    b. Fatigue, anxiety and (H) UO
    c. Jugular vein distention, peripheral edema and hepatomegaly
    d. SOB, hypoxemia, pallor

16. During an MI, hemodynamic presentation is least affected by:
    a. Pain
    b. Location of damage
    c. Residual myocardial function
    d. Extent of damage

17. During an MI, cardiogenic shock will likely occur when CI is (in L/min/m²):
    a. < 1.8
    b. < 2.2
    c. > 2.7
    d. > 4.3

18. During a Myocardial Infarction, pulmonary congestion likely begins when the PAWP exceeds (mm Hg):
    a. 12
    b. 18
    c. 25
    d. 30

19. Which combination is most likely to occur during the rewarming phase of post-op cardiac surgery?
    a. Decreased O_2 demand, Decreased CO_2 production
    b. Decreased O_2 demand, Increased CO_2 production
    c. Increased O_2 demand, Decreased CO_2 production
    d. Increased O_2 demand, Increased CO_2 production

Match the following:

Parameter		Cause
_____ 20.	Cardiogenic	a. High pressure
_____ 21.	Noncardiogenic	b. Increased permeability
_____ 22.	Hydrostatic	
_____ 23.	Neurogenic	

24. Pulmonary edema occurs when colloid osmotic pressure (COP) is:
    a. COP > PAWP
    b. COP < PAWP
    c. COP > CVP
    d. COP < CVP

25. The most common originating cause of high pressure pulmonary edema is:
    a. Intravascular volume overload
    b. Increased pulmonary venous pressure
    c. Increased LAP
    d. Increase LVEDP

26. The most common cause of non-cardiogenic pulmonary edema is:
    a. ARDS
    b. MI
    c. Stroke
    d. Renal failure

Answer the following as True (T) or False (F)

_____ 27. Permeability pulmonary edema is due to a decreased permeability of the pulmonary capillary membrane

_____ 28. The most common pulmonary complication in hospital patients is pulmonary edema

_____ 29. The most common cause of a pulmonary embolism is fat

_____ 30. A pulmonary embolism will cause an increase in deadspace ventilation

_____ 31. The hemodynamic presentation in a pulmonary embolism is usually very consistent

_____ 32. Pulmonary angiography is the most definitive test for a pulmonary embolism

Match the following:

		Parameter		Cause
_____	33.	↑ PVR	a.	Pulmonary embolus (PE)
_____	34.	Normal PVR	b.	Myocardial infarction (MI)
_____	35.	Normal PAWP		
_____	36.	↑ PAWP		

37. The first hemodynamic presentation to change in hypovolemic shock is most likely:
   a. ↓ BPdia
   b. ↑ BPdia
   c. ↓ BPsys
   d. ↑ BPsys

38. Decompensated hypovolemic shock usually occurs when volume loss exceeds:
   a. 10%
   b. 20%
   c. 30%
   d. 40%

39. Which shock is usually accompanied by bronchspasm:
    a. Anaphylactic
    b. Hypovolemic
    c. Neurogenic
    d. Septic

40. The clinical definition of cardiogenic shock includes all the following except:
    a. BPsys < 90 mm Hg
    b. Decreased HR
    c. Poor tissue perfusion
    d. UO < 20 mL/hr

41. The most common cause of cardiogenic shock is:
    a. Acute MI
    b. Arrhythmias
    c. Post-op failure
    d. Pulmonary embolism

42. Which shock type is the only one to exhibit an increased heart rate?
    a. Anaphylactic
    b. Cardiogenic
    c. Neurogenic
    d. Septic

For each of the following, indicate whether the septic shock type is Hyperdynamic (A) or Hypodynamic (B)

43. _____ Warm shock

44. _____ Cold shock

45. _____ Early phase

46. _____ Late phase

47. _____ Compensated

48. _____ Uncompensated

49. Severe aortic stenosis is indicated by an aortic valve gradient greater than (mm Hg):
    a. > 10
    b. > 20
    c. > 40
    d. > 50

50. Right Heart Failure:Backward Failure results in which of the following?
    a. Pulmonary congestion
    b. Arterial congestion
    c. Systemic perfusion deficiency
    d. Venous congestion

51. An ominous sign in aortic stenosis is:
    a. Pulmonary edema
    b. Pulmonary hypertrophy
    c. Cardiac edema
    d. Cardiac hypertrophy

CHAPTER 10
Test Questions

1. A primary pathophysiology of Acute Respiratory Distress Syndrome (ARDS) is:
   a. Overproduction of surfactant
   b. Decreased AC Membrane permeability
   c. Increased AC Membrane permeability
   d. Transudative fluid in lungs

2. Pulmonary congestion is found in which type of cardiac failure?:
   a. Left Heart: Backward Failure
   b. Left Heart: Forward Failure
   c. Right Heart: Backward Failure
   d. Right Heart: Forward Failure

3. A patient in a cardiac care unit has had about 150 mL of fluid accumulation around the heart over the last few hours. The following may be true:
   a. Cardiac impairment is likely
   b. Cardiac impairment is unlikely at this amount and time
   c. Cardiac impairment is unlikely at this time, but is likely to develop over the next days
   d. The amount of information is insufficient to predict impairment

4. Which of the following is an unlikely hemodynamic presentation for cardiac tamponade?
   a. ↑ CVP
   b. ↓ BPsys
   c. ↓ CO
   d. Normal PVR

5. A 56-year-old woman with alpha-1 antitrypsin disorder (a genetic form of COPD) is in the critical care unit. Which of the following hemodynamic parameters is most likely to reflect her chronic disease state?
   a. ↑ PVR
   b. ↓ PASP
   c. ↓ PADP
   d. Normal $S\bar{v}O_2$

6. Of critical importance in managing post-operative cardiac surgery is:
   a. Fluid resuscitation
   b. Maintaining oxygen balance
   c. Normalizing acid-base balance
   d. Rewarming as soon as possible

7. A 60-year-old female presents with shortness of breath and chest pain. The PVR is increased and PAWP is normal. Which of the following diagnoses is most likely?
   a. Myocardial infarction
   b. Decompensated hypovolemic shock
   c. Pulmonary embolus
   d. Valvular heart disease

Answer the following as True (T) or False (F)

_____ 8. PAWP is usually normal in ARDS

_____ 9. Right heart failure is the most common cause of left heart failure

_____ 10. A normal presentation of backward left heart failure is ↑ PAWP

_____ 11. A normal presentation of backward right heart failure is ↑ CVP

_____ 12. Diastolic pressure plateau is a sign of hemodynamic improvement following cardiac tamponade

_____ 13. *Pulsus paradoxicus* is common in cardiac tamponade

_____ 14. COPD patients often have decreased lung zones 1 and 2

_____ 15. During an MI, pulmonary congestion will begin at a PAWP > 30 mm Hg

_____ 16. Oxygen supply/demand balance is the major determinant of post-op morbidity and mortality

_____ 17. Normal colloid osmotic pressure (COP) is 6-15 mm Hg

_____ 18. Pulmonary edema occurs when COP > PAWP

_____ 19. Pulmonary edema's second stage of progression is interstitial edema

_____ 20. The most common type of pulmonary edema is permeability pulmonary edema

_____ 21. The most common cause of high pressure pulmonary edema is left ventricular dysfunction

_____ 22. The most definitive test for pulmonary embolism is a lung ventilation / perfusion scan

_____ 23. The two types of hypovolemic shock are hypodynamic and hyperdynamic

_____ 24. Blood pressure is the most sensitive and accurate indicator of hypovolemic shock

_____ 25. Cardiogenic shock is the only shock resulting in a decreased heart rate

_____ 26. Hypodynamic phase is the later phase of septic shock

_____ 27. Moderate aortic stenosis is usually asymptomatic

_____ 28. The most likely hemodynamic presentation in mitral stenosis is increased LAP

_____ 29. Aortic regurgitation may be either compensated or uncompensated

_____ 30. The body's first compensation for mitral stenosis is an increased cardiac output

_____ 31. In mitral regurgitation the best indicator of LVEDP is PAWP

1. A 6-year-old arrives in the Emergency Department in reported anaphylactic shock after consuming peanuts with a known severe allergy. Build a case study - this is a powerful way to learn. Give actual findings and values. Avoid giving ranges or generic information (such as "difficulty breathing" - give details about what that would look like). Use the following to guide you:

    a. What clinical manifestations would you expect to see at this point?

    b. Describe the hemodynamic presentation you would expect to see.

    c. Based upon the information you provided in a and b, what management steps would you recommend (be specific.)?

2. You are asked to provide a "respiratory consult" on a 66-year-old female, 5'2", 96 kg. She is currently on a nonrebreather, running at 12 L/min. Chest X-ray shows opacities throughout the lung fields. The following information has also been gathered:

HR	112 bpm		RR	36 breaths/min
SpO₂	88%		BP	88/56 mm Hg

pH	7.32
PaCO₂	51 mm Hg
PaO₂	52 mm Hg
HCO₃	25 mEq/L

CO	5.2 L/min		PAP	18/6 mm Hg
PVR	310 dynes-sec-cm⁻⁵		PCWP	13 mm Hg
CVP	5 mm Hg			

Based upon the information provided, what diagnosis is most likely? Give evidence for your diagnosis.

Answer Keys

Chapter 1
Review Questions

1.	b	11.	d	21.	c
2.	j	12.	h	22.	g
3.	i	13.	j	23.	j
4.	g	14.	a	24.	f
5.	h	15.	f	25.	h
6.	d	16.	i	26.	a
7.	f	17.	b	27.	d
8.	c	18.	g	28.	e
9.	e	19.	c	29.	b
10.	a	20.	e	30.	i

31.	c	41.	f	51.	d
32.	i	42.	b	52.	b
33.	b	43.	h	53.	a
34.	e	44.	j	54.	f
35.	a	45.	c	55.	e
36.	h	46.	g	56.	c
37.	d	47.	d	57.	g
38.	f	48.	a	58.	h
39.	j	49.	e	59.	e
40.	g	50.	i	60.	i

61.	a	71.	h	81.	e
62.	d	72.	b	82.	b
63.	c	73.	i	83.	h
64.	j	74.	a	84.	g
65.	b	75.	f	85.	f
66.	g	76.	g	86.	j
67.	f	77.	d	87.	i
68.	c	78.	d	88.	d
69.	e	79.	c	89.	a
70.	j	80.	a	90.	j

91.	h	101.	f	111.	a
92.	i	102.	a	112.	c
93.	b	103.	e	113.	b
94.	f	104.	c	114.	d
95.	c	105.	d	115.	i
96.	e	106.	b	116.	j
97.	g	107.	e	117.	h
98.	i	108.	f	118.	c
99.	g	109.	h	119.	a
100.	h	110.	g	120.	i

121.	j	131.	e
122.	b	132.	f
123.	f	133.	b
124.	e	134.	a
125.	d	135.	h
126.	g	136.	i
127.	d		
128.	c		
129.	g		
130.	j		

Chapter 1
Test Questions

1.	c	11.	d	21.	c
2.	b	12.	h	22.	a
3.	c	13.	f	23.	c
4.	a	14.	b	24.	b
5.	d	15.	i	25.	c
6.	c	16.	a	26.	c
7.	b	17.	g	27.	b
8.	b	18.	j	28.	a
9.	a	19.	c	29.	d
10.	e	20.	c	30.	d

31.	d	41.	h
32.	b	42.	k
33.	b	43.	b
34.	a	44.	e
35.	d	45.	j
36.	f	46.	F
37.	g	47.	T
38.	i	48.	T
39.	a	49.	T
40.	c	50.	T

Chapter 2
Review Questions

1. a. oxygen
   b. nutrients
   c. equal to the need
   d. maintain a balance between the supply and demand

		11.	b	21.	c
2.	↑	12.	b	22.	b
3.	↓	13.	b	23.	f
4.	↓	14.	c	24.	b
5.	↓	15.	b	25.	d
6.	↓	16.	a	26.	f
7.	↓	17.	d	27.	b
8.	↓	18.	a	28.	c
9.	↑	19.	d	29.	a
10.	a	20.	e	30.	e

31.	MvO2	41.	CO	51.	F
32.	MDO2	42.	CO	52.	T
33.	MvO2	43.	CI	53.	F
34.	MvO2	44.	CO	54.	T
35.	MDO2	45.	CI	55.	T
36.	T	46.	F	56.	F
37.	T	47.	T	57.	T
38.	F	48.	F	58.	T
39.	T	49.	T	59.	F
40.	T	50.	T	60.	F

61.	F	71.	F
62.	F	72.	F
63.	F	73.	T
64.	F		
65.	T		
66.	T		
67.	T		
68.	T		
69.	F		
70.	T		

Chapter 2
Test Questions

1.	d	11.	a	21.	i
2.	c	12.	e	22.	f
3.	b	13.	a	23.	g
4.	d	14.	e	24.	a
5.	a	15.	c	25.	d
6.	c	16.	d	26.	e
7.	b	17.	b	27.	c
8.	c	18.	b	28.	b
9.	a	19.	h	29.	f
10.	d	20.	b	30.	d

31.	a	41.	b	51.	a
32.	c	42.	c	52.	c
33.	e	43.	b	53.	a
34.	b	44.	c	54.	d
35.	d	45.	a	55.	a
36.	c	46.	b		
37.	b	47.	b		
38.	c	48.	b		
39.	a	49.	c		
40.	a	50.	d		

Chapter 3
Review Questions

1.	a	11.	T	21.	F
2.	c	12.	F	22.	F
3.	b	13.	F	23.	↑
4.	d	14.	T	24.	↓
5.	a	15.	F	25.	↓
6.	b	16.	T	26.	↑
7.	d	17.	T	27.	↓
8.	c	18.	F	28.	↑
9.	a	19.	F		
10.	T	20.	T		

Chapter 3
Test Questions

1.	b
2.	d
3.	b
4.	d
5.	a
6.	c
7.	b
8.	a
9.	d
10.	c

Chapter 4
Review Questions

1. b
2. a
3. b
4. d
5. c

Chapter 5
Review Questions

#		#		#	
1.	T	11.	b	21.	c
2.	T	12.	a	22.	f
3.	F	13.	d	23.	b
4.	T	14.	a	24.	d
5.	T	15.	b	25.	a
6.	e	16.	d		
7.	c	17.	c		
8.	a	18.	a		
9.	b	19.	c		
10.	d	20.	e		

Chapter 5
Test Questions

#		#		#	
1.	b	11.	e	21.	a
2.	d	12.	a	22.	a
3.	a	13.	f		
4.	c	14.	c		
5.	b	15.	b		
6.	a	16.	d		
7.	c	17.	c		
8.	b	18.	a		
9.	d	19.	d		
10.	b	20.	c		

Chapter 6
Review Questions

1.	b	11.	T	21.	↑
2.	c	12.	T	22.	↑
3.	d	13.	F	23.	↓
4.	c	14.	F		
5.	a	15.	F		
6.	b	16.	F		
7.	T	17.	F		
8.	F	18.	F		
9.	T	19.	↓		
10.	F	20.	↑		

Chapter 6
Test Questions

1.	b	11.	c
2.	d	12.	b
3.	a	13.	F
4.	c	14.	T
5.	d	15.	F
6.	a		
7.	a		
8.	a		
9.	a		
10.	a		

ANSWER KEYS

Chapter 7
Review Questions

1.	b	11.	T	21.	F
2.	d	12.	F	22.	F
3.	c	13.	a	23.	F
4.	b	14.	d	24.	M
5.	a	15.	c	25.	D
6.	F	16.	b	26.	M
7.	F	17.	d	27.	D
8.	F	18.	a	28.	M
9.	T	19.	T	29.	D
10.	F	20.	T	30.	D

31.	M	41.	a	51.	1
32.	M	42.	d	52.	1
33.	M	43.	↓	53.	2
34.	D	44.	↑	54.	1
35.	D	45.	↑	55.	3
36.	c	46.	↓	56.	1
37.	b	47.	c	57.	2
38.	d	48.	d	58.	3
39.	b	49.	b	59.	d
40.	b	50.	3	60.	T

61.	T	71.	T
62.	T	72.	T
63.	T	73.	T
64.	T	74.	F
65.	F		
66.	F		
67.	b		
68.	b		
69.	F		
70.	F		

Chapter 7
Test Questions

1.	T	11.	a	21.	a
2.	T	12.	a		
3.	F	13.	c		
4.	F	14.	d		
5.	F	15.	a		
6.	T	16.	a		
7.	T	17.	a		
8.	F	18.	c		
9.	d	19.	d		
10.	c	20.	c		

Chapter 8
Review Questions

1. c
2. g
3. a
4. e
5. d
6. f
7. b
8. d
9. c
10. d

Chapter 9
Review Questions

1. b
2. a
3. c
4. b
5. d
6. a
7. T
8. F
9. F
10. T

Chapter 8
Test Questions

1. b
2. c
3. d
4. c
5. a

Chapter 9
Test Questions

1. a
2. a
3. a
4. a
5. d
6. a
7. c